By D

SCIATICA RELIEVED

Home Exercises and Tips That Actually Work

SCIATICA RELIEVED

Home Exercises and Tips That Actually Work

Disclaimer

Not all sciatica back pain is similar. The nature of pain, their causes, and effects all differ from one case to another and so do their treatment plan. Though most of the sciatica sufferer would benefit from the tips and exercises described here, but still, this book is not a replacement of professional medical consultation, diagnosis, and investigation. We have included precautions and warnings in each step of the journey of the sciatica case. If you find symptoms worsening or exercises not responding, you must seek professional medical advice at the earliest.

Image Credit

Vertebral column:

By Servier Medical Art by Servier, https://smart.servier.com/

Intervertebral disc:

By Servier Medical Art by Servier, https://smart.servier.com/

Disc hernia:

By Servier Medical Art by Servier, https://smart.servier.com/

Piriformis syndrome:

By Servier Medical Art by Servier, https://smart.servier.com/

Sciatic nerve:

Blausen.com staff (2014). "Medical gallery of Blausen Medical 2014". WikiJournal of Medicine 1 (2). DOI:10.15347/wjm/2014.010. ISSN 2002-4436. [CC BY 3.0 (creativecommons.org/licenses/by/3.0)]

Forward

As an Occupational Therapist, I know Sunit Sanjay Ekka from since last 16 years. He was my student at SVNIRTAR (Swami Vivekananda National Institute of Rehabilitation and Research, a Government of India institution under Ministry of Social Justice and Empowerment). I appreciate his dedication to his patient. I can see his instinct to bring positive changes in the lives of his patients. His knowledge will surely guide you towards the proper direction of getting rehabilitation from your pain, suffering, and disability.

Sunil Mokashi,
Ex-Head of the Department, Occupational Therapy.
SVNIRTAR (Govt of India)

Table of content

Preface

I am a physiotherapist and have been working with back pain cases from since last 14 years. During this period I have helped numerous back pain cases diagnosed with sciatica.

In my experience sciatica is the major cause of back pain and of course, it is most debilitating too. They usually come to me after receiving initial medication. Going through their reports reveals that analgesics are the main prescribed medicine. They are also advised for bed rest.

Analgesics gives them only momentarily relief. Pain and disability affect their job and profession which is the major cause of their frustration.

Sciatica pain and disability vary from mild to severe condition.

Mild conditions, from here by we call it "subacute phase", are those who have a complaint of back pain with a burning sensation on the leg. They have difficulty in walking but can manage their daily chores.

Severe sciatica conditions, we call it as "acute phase", are bedridden and go through severe pain. A slightest of lower body movement or twist is enough to elicit flare unbearable pain. For the several days of bed rest is helpful. If things get worse, an acute phase can also exhibit signs of paraparesis and lower leg weakness.

This book would be of great help for a person with sciatica in the subacute phase. It is equally helpful for an acute phase sciatica sufferer, who can refer it for many effective pain-relieving tips. This book has some invaluable tips for acute sciatica which I myself have applied to many of my patients and prevent them from surgery. Hope this could also help you as a severe sciatica sufferer.

Let me point it down an important thing before we begin, the road to recovery is not going to be a smooth ride. Someday you may feel as if the pain is almost gone and the other day pain may flare-up.

But, if the journey has begun it has to reach its pain-free destination. The reader of the book should be aware that the treatment process of sciatica includes a combination of Physiotherapy, electrotherapy, manual therapy, and home exercises.

This book will cover every treatment aspect that you might go through but will mainly focus on precaution home tips and the most important exercise.

With this, I would like to wish all sciatica sufferer my best wishes and speedy recovery.

How to use this book

Sciatica in its worst form "acute phase" can make you bedridden. In a little milder form "subacute phase" it allows you to walk but with pain and difficulty.

You will find lots of information on the Internet regarding sciatica and its exercises. Please keep in mind that not all exercises are beneficial. The particular exercise that fits for the milder form of sciatica could be beyond the capacity for a severe sciatica sufferer. In fact, it may result in an increase in pain.

Exercises have to be carefully chosen. It varies with different severity and pain condition. The treatment approach also changes with the improvement of pain.

This is why we have carefully picked up the best exercises for each different phase. We have tried to describe a journey of sciatica sufferer through this diagram.

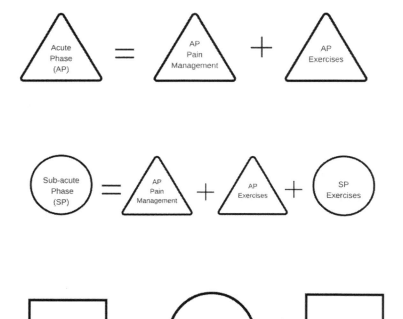

Each of the shapes signifies different phases of sciatica and their corresponding pain management program and exercises program.

- ❏ Triangle shape = Phase of severe sciatica.
- ❏ Circle shape = Phase of mild sciatica.
- ❏ Square = Rehabilitation phase.

Observe how the exercise of the acute phase is being repeated on the subacute phase but is excluded in the rehabilitation phase

The journey of sciatica sufferer can begin from any of the phases, but regardless of its starting point it always travels in the upside-down direction.

Not yet clear?

Ok, let's try to understand with an example. For which we have to go to our next chapter "the story of Mr. Sethi" and come back again here.

In our story Mr. Sethy was suffering from subacute sciatica, so his journey starts from the circular phase traveling down to square phase.

Though your doctor is the best person to decide which stage/ phase of sciatica you are in, but in the next chapter, we will extensively discuss in detail each and every phase. Reading further could help you to some extent in understanding your pain and its phase.

Story of Mr. Sethy

Seriously! This could be your story. A story of his journey from painful sciatica to a pain-free life.

L et me tell you a story about Mr. Sethy. One of my successfully treated patient and he was back in his work within 2 weeks.

Your case may not be exactly the same but you can get some inspiration out of his journey.
When he came to me, he was emotionally down and physically in pain.

"If physiotherapy won't work I may need to go for spinal surgery," told Mr. Sethy. He further added that his neurosurgeon has advised to "go physiotherapy for at least a month and let me review it again after a month".

He came to me with lots of hope and I did not want him to go empty-handed. With all the dedication, professionalism and prayer, our 8 months long journey begins.

Mr. Sethy is a well-known successful owner of the printing press of the town. Though he has the number of employees working on the press, often he himself has to get engaged to compensate for the staff shortage.

His work usually involves cross sitting on the floor and arranging stacks of paper for the final trimming and binding to turn a stack of papers into a book. Each stack would weigh around 5 to 10 Kg and often he has to lift the stack manually from one point to another point.

"It was a busy afternoon and a customer's target was to be fulfilled," told Mr. Sethy to me. In an arbiter attempt to lift a stack of paper that would weigh around 10kg he bends forward. The very moment when he lifts the stack slightly away from the ground he felt a pinch like pain on the back.

"Before I could make out what happened, I found myself locked in and bending position," said Mr. Sethy, "and any attempt to erect myself in myself was very painful".

Escorted by their staff, he went for bed rest in his house upstairs. The following day he managed to visit his physician, the physician prescribed him analgesics and referred him to a Neurosurgeon.

Following is the important point to be noted:

- He himself is overweight.
- His profession demands him to sit cross-legged for long hours.
- The pain started instantaneously when he bent forward to lift a weight.

The story goes further like this. The Neurologist advised him for a detailed investigation and suggested a lower back MRI.

Before any final diagnosis could be made, he was under analgesics and bed rest. He was also prescribed a lumbar support brace. After two days when the MRI report was delivered and it was diagnosed to be L4- L5 lumbar disc bulge. A serious internal back injury.

He visited me after a week. Till then his acute pain was reduced and could walk with little difficulty. When he came to me his body was bent at lower back to the right side.

He described his pain in the following way:

1. Pain in the low back with pulling or tingling sensation running down the leg
2. Unable to walk or stand straight.
3. Walking is difficult as it produces painful pulling sensation to the left leg.

We carried out rigorous physiotherapy for almost 8 months. Within 2 weeks he was back to his work. But it took almost 8 months to fully rehabilitate him.

His neurosurgeon told "If you can walk, carry on with work, then what's the necessity of surgery", Mr. Sethy smiled and said, "I will surely do few exercises for the rest of my life and follow few precautions".

Are you really suffering from sciatica?

U nderstanding your back pain is important. It will help you in distinguishing between good exercise and bad exercise.

The Internet is flooded with information about sciatica exercises, but one should be careful that not all exercises are valid. In fact, the authenticity of the source itself is in the question. Every third person, even though not a qualified health professional, claims himself /herself a guru of sciatica treatment.

Remember, a wrong exercise will do more bad to your back pain than anything else. After 14 years of professional dedication and successfully dealing with back pain, I have come up with a few simple steps to recognize the type of back pain you might be suffering from.

These steps are very simple. It can give you a broader picture of the actual problem on your back. But do keep in mind that that this is not a replacement for professional medical investigation.

So before moving ahead, let us first discuss types of back pain.

To simplify it, back pain can be broadly classified under two subheadings.

1: Localised back pain.
2: Back pain with radiation to lower leg.

Localized back pain

In localized back pain, the pain is only felt in and around the lower back. The person complains of pain and tenderness only around the lower back region.

The localized back pain could be due to muscle spasm or trigger points.
Usually, this type of pain is very old (muscle spasm is an exception, which develops instantaneously) they do not start all of a sudden and it develops slowly with the time.

If I ask for the exact day when you started this back pain perhaps you may recollect it. This is because this type of pain is usually very old they develop slowly with time.

Some of the important cause of such pain is:

- Sitting habitually in the wrong posture.
- Often associated with professions like a truck driver, whose profession involves long hours of driving in a single sitting position.

Back pain with radiation to lower leg

In this type, pain in addition to the lower back is also felt (referred to) on the lower leg. It means the sufferer will have low back pain and also complaint of pain (with burning and pulling sensation) radiating down to the legs. It could be on one single leg or both the leg simultaneously.

This book is only concerned with this type of back pain. Pain radiating to the leg is a red flag indicating possible internal neuronal involvement. Most probably it could be due to sciatica.

Guide to recognizing your back pain.

First, try to observe your pain and ask yourself these questions.

1. Do I feel pain only on the back?
2. Is there any kind of pain other than the lower back pain?
3. Am I feeling any pulling sensation or tingling sensation on my legs?
4. Do I feel uncomfortable during walking or standing on my legs?

If you have come up with the answers, then again ask these questions.

1. When did my pain start?
2. Am I able to remember the exact day when my pain started?
3. How did it start?
4. Did it start on its own or while lifting a heavyweight, during jumping or twisting (try to associate incident that could have triggered your pain)?

Note down your answers in a piece of paper. Try to evaluate and compare it with the probable answers given below.

You might come across one among the two following answers.

1. You only have pain concentrated to your lower back and unable to recollect the exact day or incident which triggered the pain.
2. The second condition is, you have pain on your back and you also feel pulling sensation or painful tingling sensation on the lower legs. It could be a right leg or left leg and you can easily associate with the incident. The incident could be a jerk, twisting, jumping and lifting heavyweight or anything like this.

So what's your answer?

If your answer is the first one, then you are on a safer side. This pain can easily be managed with a few effective tips. We have got some most effective pain-relieving tips and techniques in our chapter, you can apply it and see your pain vanishing in no time.

But if the second point is your answer, then it's a matter of concern. You might be suffering from a neurological problem known as sciatica.

Once again, let me remind you that this is not a replacement for professional medical investigation. You should take professional help to get fully diagnosed and pinpoint the cause of pain.

Basic anatomy of the spine

The human body is an amazing engineering masterpiece. Our upper trunk is like heavy log supported over the lower back and two limbs. When we sit, stand, walk or run, look how beautifully it is balanced in an erect position against all forces and gravity.

While maintaining its stable and erect posture, it is also flexible, so that we can bend forward, backward and can twist. Have you ever wondered how is it possible?

It is possible because of the vertebral column. Vertebral column also known as spinal column is made up of vertebral bodies arranged one above the other. Imagine bricks kept one over the other, in the same way, the vertebral body is arranged and held in place by ligaments connecting and holding each other(1).

At its upper end, the vertebral column articulates with the skull base and thereby supports the skull. The inferior part of the vertebral column articulates on each side, with the corresponding hip bone. The two hip bones are united anteriorly at the pubic symphysis to form the pelvic girdle.

The human body has a total number of 33 vertebrae.

These are:

- Cervical spine: 7 vertebrae (C1–C7)
- Thoracic spine: 12 vertebrae (T1–T12)
- Lumbar spine: 5 vertebrae (L1–L5)
- Sacrum: 5 (fused) vertebrae (S1–S5)
- Coccyx: 4 (3–5) (fused) vertebrae (Tailbone).

On the posterior side of the vertebral column, there is a canal-like structure. This Canal like structure is called a spinal canal. The spinal cord which originates from the brain passes through this spinal canal down till L5.

Intervertebral disc

Between every two consecutive vertebral bodies is present intervertebral disc. The intervertebral disc (Figure 5) is the principal bond between adjacent vertebral bodies. There are 23 intervertebral discs in all, the first being located between C2 and C3 vertebral bodies and the last disc being situated at the lumbosacral junction.

Each intervertebral disc is made up of two structures: an outer lamellated (multi-layered) fibrous ring termed annulus fibrosus and a gelatinous inner zone termed the nucleus pulposus(1). The inner nucleus pulposus is a soft jelly-like structure that functions as a shock absorber.

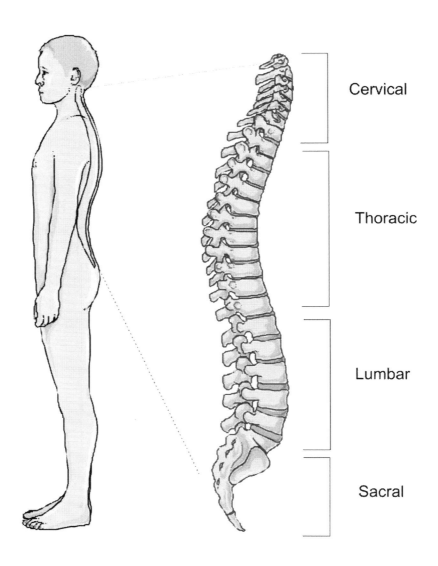

Cervical

Thoracic

Lumbar

Sacral

Understanding Sciatica

The feeling of electrical shock firing on the back of the leg. As if pinpricks in my heels. The debilitating pains of sciatica made your life come to a grinding halt.

D o you remember that *pinch* like feel on the low back that started your sciatica pain? The *pinch* turned into pain with the feeling as if electric shock firing on the back of the leg. One of my clients described "as if pinpricks in my heels, it's painful while stair climbing".

The sciatica sufferer often describes a feeling of pulling sensation on the leg, "I just loved to knock me off my feet, and force me to sit down at the most opportune times I could find" described a sciatica sufferer.

A painful event that turned an otherwise simple daily activity into a painful challenge. You can no more help your wife with household work, going shopping, loading and unloading have become a nightmare. Forget about playing with your kids. When you sit on motorbike you tilt yourself to one side of the buttock while trying to keep straight to avoid pain.

As the days pass by, the condition gets worse with feel tingling sensation and numbness on leg and feet. You went to your doctor and you were diagnosed with a serious case of sciatica.

Epidemiology of sciatica

Sciatica is a relatively common condition with a lifetime incidence varying from 13% to 40%.
A number of environmental and inherent factors thought to influence the development of sciatica have been studied, including gender, body habitus, parity, age, genetic factors, occupation, and environmental factors(2).

Few of the important takeaway from British Journal of Anaesthesia:

- Incident of sciatica is related to age - peaks in the fifth decade.
- The majority of disc hernia occurs at L4-L5 or L5-S1 level. With advancing age, there appears to be a relatively increased incidence of herniation at L3-L4 or even L2-L3 level.
- Physical activity associated with occupation has also been shown to influence the incidence of sciatica. Like a carpenter, machine operator, diving.
- Male is more affected than female

What is sciatica?

The name sciatica is commonly given to any painful neuralgic condition that starts from the buttock and travels down along the course of the great sciatic nerve. The ancient Greeks were familiar with sciatic neuralgia and used the term 'sciatica', to describe pains or 'ischias' felt around the hip or thigh(2).

According to *web*MD "sciatica is a pain, tingling or numbness produced by an irritation of the nerve root that leads to the sciatic nerve".

Let me simplify it, sciatica simply means a problem with the sciatic nerve. But, the question is what is this sciatic nerve, from where they originate and where it goes?

The sciatic nerve is the longest and thickest nerve in the human body that originates from the pelvic region. The fourth and fifth lumbar nerve roots and the first two sacral nerve roots join in the lumbosacral plexus to form the peroneal and tibial nerves that leave the pelvis in an ensheathed single trunk as the sciatic nerve, the largest nerve in the body(3).

They leave the lumbar (low back) region passes through buttocks and travels down the thighs and backside of the leg to end near the sole of the feet.

Disturbances anywhere along the course of the sciatic nerve can give rise to sciatica, but the most common areas are at the sites of disk rupture and osteoarthritic change — at the L4–L5 and L5–S1 levels and, less frequently, the L3–L4 level — where there is usually compression of the root below the corresponding disk(3).

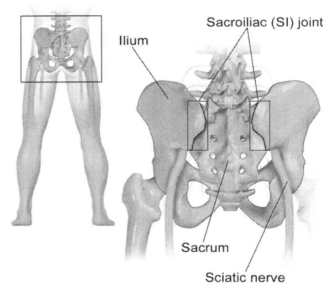

Sacroiliac Joint

Symptoms of sciatica

A person with sciatica typically complains of pain coming suddenly or sometimes gradually. They will describe the pain as burning or sharp shooting electric shock-like pain radiates from the outer sides of buttocks to the thigh and lower leg.
Low back pain of variable severity accompanies sciatica but is not a consistent feature. Aching in the L5–S1 area or in the upper sacroiliac joint is common with disk rupture. Increased back and sciatic pain with coughing, sneezing, straining, or other forms of the Valsalva maneuver suggests disk rupture(3).

They have a complaint of difficulty in daily work. I have compiled some of the common complaint in this pictorial form.

1: Pain during brushing teeth.

When brushing teeth you need to slightly bend forward eliciting pain.

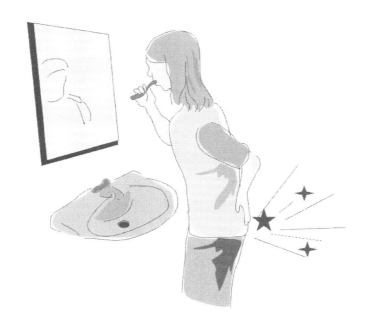

2: Riding motorbike/ scooter a painful experience.

Often you may tilt to one side to avoid pain

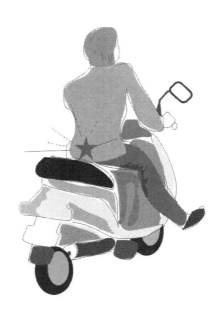

3: Lifting your baby (any object) is a struggle.

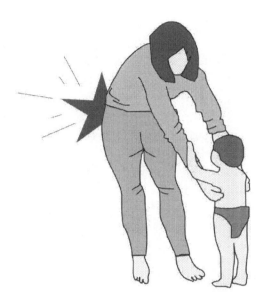

There are other symptoms described below in a bullet point.

- The peculiarity of sciatica pain is that the pain starts from the lower back to the buttocks and down the legs in one particular line along the nerve pathway.
- Pain could be varying from a mild ache to a sharp, electric shock-like or burning in nature.
- Constant pain in one leg making it difficult for the patient to sit or stand for a prolonged period of time.
- Feeling of numbness, tingling and weakness of the muscles in the affected leg.
- In severe cases of sciatica, the patient may experience trouble in controlling the bowels or bladder movement.

What went wrong in your back

Sciatica is the compression and irritation of the sciatic nerve. Sciatic nerve compression can occur in three places. First is, when this nerve is just branching out of the spinal cord, second is when it is coming out of the spinal canal through the neural canal. In the third condition, it gets compressed away from the vertebral column.

There could be two causes of sciatic nerve compression, spinal cause, and non-spinal cause.

Spinal cause includes

1. Lumbar disc bulging and hernia of L4, L5, and S1 root.
2. Spine degeneration
3. Spondylolisthesis.
4. Spinal stenosis: The narrowing of the spinal canal puts pressure on the sciatic nerve and causes sciatica.

Non-spinal cause

1. Piriformis syndrome
2. Spondylolisthesis
3. Sacroiliac dysfunction.
4. In rare circumstances, the sciatic nerve can be compressed by a tumor or damaged by a disease such as long-term diabetes.

Sciatica due to disk rupture and degenerative spine disease is more common than sciatica due to all nonspinal causes taken together(3). And piriformis syndrome is the most common cause among non-spinal cause.

In the next section, we will try to understand what actually happens in disc rupture/ hernia which will help us to understand sciatica better.

Let's try to understand it through a diagram and proceed to next chapter on disc bulge

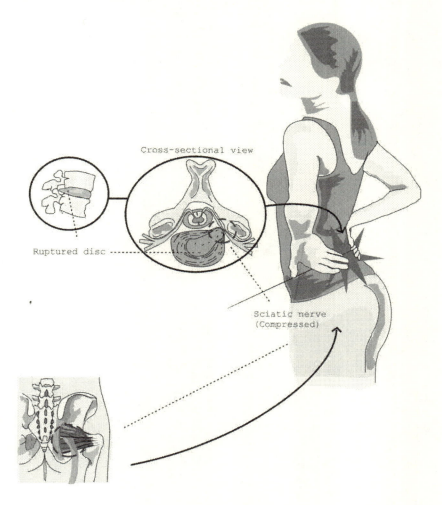

Cross-sectional view

Ruptured disc ---------

Sciatic nerve
(Compressed)

Disc bulge/ Disc hernia/ Slip disc

The most important and most common cause of sciatica. But you too can get out of it without surgery.

A disc bulge is also known by other names such as prolapsed intervertebral disc, disc hernia, slip disc.

Contrary to the belief that disc is displaced from its original place, actually in a slipped disc, the intervertebral disc gets punctured. The puncture or tear in disc causes jelly-like material to come out and put pressure on the nerve that is passing by.

To understand this we need to understand the basics of intervertebral disc anatomy.

Intervertebral disc anatomy

Our backbone is made up of the vertebral column. The human vertebral column has a total number of 31 vertebral bodies and between each vertebral body, there is an intervertebral disc that links them together.

Their major role is mechanical, as they constantly transmit loads arising from body weight and muscle activity through the spinal column(4). They provide flexibility, observe that whenever we bend forward or backward, we twist sideways, rotate or jump this intervertebral disc acts as a shock absorber.

They are approximately 7 to 10 mm thick and 4 cm in diameter (anterior-posterior plane) in the lumbar region of the spine.6,7 The intervertebral discs are complex structures that consist of a thick outer ring of fibrous cartilage termed the annulus fibrosus, which surrounds a more gelatinous core known as the nucleus pulposus(4). This nucleus pulposus jelly-like material and is made up of 80% of water.

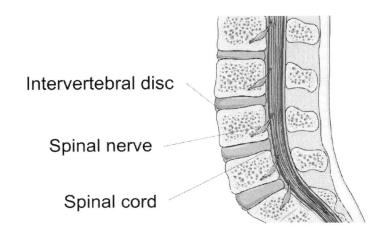

Intervertebral disc

Spinal nerve

Spinal cord

The importance of the intervertebral disc can be compared with a shock absorber in our motorbike or car. Imagine what will happen if the shock absorber from our vehicles is removed. The person traveling in such a vehicle is sure to sustain internal damage on the lower back. Let alone the traveler, the vehicle itself will get internal damages.

In the same way, intervertebral disc absorbs all the shock from the ground exerted during jumping or running and protects our bones and internal organs from damage.

What goes wrong in a slipped disc?

The intervertebral disc has a central nucleus pulposus with soft jelly encircled by a stiff fibrous outer ring known as annulus fibrosus. In prolapsed disc/ disc herniation, the outer annulus fibrosus ring gets ruptured & a fissure is developed over time. Resulting in central jelly-like material to bulge out, in severe cases, it may even leak out through fissure causing a pressure/ compression of the nerve.

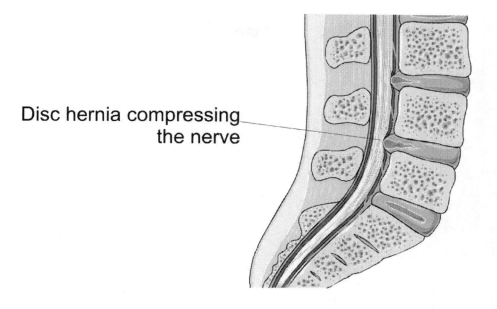

Disc hernia compressing the nerve

Herniated part of disc compressing the spinal nerve

The disc lesions can be classified as Contained or Herniated. The progression of disc degeneration can further be classified as follows(4):

Grade 1/ Disc bulging: Annular tearing confined to the inner region of the annulus fibrosis. In grade 2, a tear or fissure becomes visible. It extends from the nucleus radially into the inner one-third of the annulus fibrosus.

Grade 2/ Disc protrusion: In this condition, annular tears have completely disrupted the disc architecture but do not affect the outer contour of the annulus. The entire annulus is disrupted. There is no leakage of injected dye on discography from the disc, nor bulging nor protrusion of the disc. There is no compressive effect on the corresponding nerve root. Many of these patients with complaints of lower back pain, which may travel into the lower limb and even past the knee into the lower leg and foot.

Grade 3/ Disc extrusion: In this situation, tears have completely disrupted the annulus fibrosus and deformed the contour of the posterior portion of the disc. By this stage, there is a complete tear of fibrous exterior and the soft jelly nucleus comes out. As a result, it compresses the spinal nerve with even more pressure resulting in an acute painful condition.

Grade 4/ Disc sequestration: The extruded part of the disc when it becomes free and detached we call it a disc sequestration stage. The detached part of the nucleus pulposus lies in the epidural space. This is the stage where surgery remains the only option of treatment. So, we will not discuss the sequestration stage int his book.

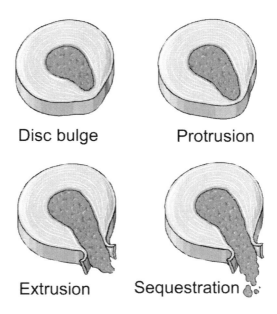

Disc bulge   Protrusion

Extrusion   Sequestration

Bulging or protrusion of disc can further occur in different directions
- Central disc bulge.
- Left side disc bulge.
- Right side disc bulge.

In central disc bulge, the right side sciatic nerve and the left side are equally compressed. The person complains of pain in both the leg. On the left side or right side disc bulge, the sufferer complains of pain on the corresponding leg.

Piriformis syndrome

A painful condition on the outer side of buttocks. A lesser-known and often ignored, but important cause of sciatica.

P eople often associate sciatica pain to prolapsed intervertebral disc/ disc herniation. There is another cause of sciatica which is fairly common and often overlooked. This is piriformis syndrome.

It can be best described by pain on one side (sometimes both the side) of the buttock in association with a backache. The piriformis syndrome has been attributed to compression of the sciatic nerve underlying the piriformis muscle, which stabilizes and serves as an external rotator of the hip(3).

To have a better picture, let us cover some basics of piriformis muscle anatomy. But before we proceed, let me tell clarify that the clinical feature of piriformis syndrome is similar to sciatica caused by the disc herniation.

Relevant anatomy of piriformis

In the term "piriformis syndrome", the piriformis is a muscle. Piriformis muscle is situated deep on the sides of the buttock. The piriformis is a flat, pear-shaped muscle located in the gluteal region of the hip/proximal thigh.

The piriformis muscle originates from the anterior sacrum and sacroiliac joint, passes transversely through the greater sciatic foramen via the sciatic notch, and inserts on the greater trochanter.

The piriformis muscle rotates the femur during the extension of the hip and abducts the femur during flexion of the hip. As it passes through and nearly completely fills the greater sciatic foramen, the muscle divides the foramen into a superior and inferior segment(5).

The sciatic nerve generally exits the pelvis inferior to the piriformis muscle, however, variations do occur and the entire never may pass superior to or through the muscle. In other variations, the sciatic nerve may be split into its major divisions which may lie on either side of the piriformis, or one division can pass through the muscle with the other division above or below the muscle belly(5).

Now, look at the picture which will make the concept clear.

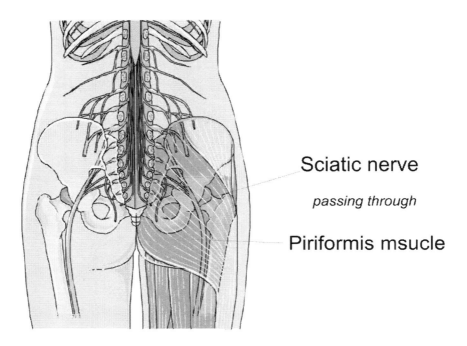

Sciatic nerve

passing through

Piriformis msucle

What goes wrong in the piriformis syndrome?

Now that we know sciatic nerve passes through the piriformis muscle, what will happen if it gets stuck between the muscle fiber? Yes, this is what happens in piriformis syndrome, the great sciatic nerve gets compressed inside the piriformis muscle.

Compression or irritation of the sciatic nerve can occur when the piriformis muscle becomes inflamed, has spasms, or becomes tight. Typically, this results from overuse, prolonged sitting, and activities such as rowing in the sitting position. In addition, weak hip abductor muscles, such as the gluteals, combined with tight adductors, increase the risk if they do not engage regularly(6).

The compressed nerve produces pain and current /tingling like sensation on all the parts where they travel (back of thigh and leg).

Phases of sciatica

Symptoms, exercises, home tips, your physiotherapist's role, everything about every phase.

S ciatica may begin either suddenly with physical activity or slowly. Sciatic pain has aching and sharp components and radiates along a broad line from the middle or lower buttock and travels down the leg(3).

- In L5 nerve root compression pain proceeds posterolaterally in the thigh.
- It proceeds via posterior in cases of compression of S1.
- With L4 compression, the pain is anterolateral in the thigh and maybe misattributed to hip disease.

Low back pain of variable severity accompanies sciatica but is not a consistent
feature. Aching in the L5–S1 area or in the upper sacroiliac joint is common with
disk rupture(3).

For ease of understanding and managing, sciatica is categorized under three phases. This is based on the severity of pain and disability. Disability means whether the person is bedridden or is able to move/ walk. Is he able to walk easily or with pain? What's the underlying cause? Whether its 3rd stage hernia or something else

Taking all this into consideration we have three phases.

1. Acute phase.
2. Subacute phase.
3. Rehabilitation phase.

Remember our triangle, circular, square shape designating each different phase.

In the next coming chapters, we will dive deeper into each phase, its clinical feature, precaution, home treatment tips, the role of your physiotherapist, we will cover everything.

Go through each chapter carefully, follow the advice and warning signal carefully for the best result.

So, let's get started.

Acute Phase

The most painful phase, rest is best at this stage. But, these tips can help to manage pain at home. This is how Physiotherapists can help you.

The acute phase is the most painful phase of all, the sufferer goes through severe pain. I have seen patients with acute sciatica often describing their pain as "so unbearable that it feels as if it's better to have my legs separated from the body". The magnitude of pain could be guessed from this statement.

In this stage, pain is more apparent on legs than the lower back. The sharp shooting pain starts from the lower back and travels down the backside of the leg through the back of the thigh.

The patient usually comes to the OPD or physiotherapy department carried by their relative on a stretcher. A slightest of movement or twist at the lower back is enough to elicit the pain.

Main cause of acute sciatica is stage 3 disc degeneration. In this stage, the disc protrusion or damage to the disc is irreversible. It protrudes to a point where chances of rearrangement of protruded part of disc become minimal, leaving the surgery as the only option. But, sometimes it has as been found that taking bed rest can reduce some acuteness.

In this chapter, we will cover how we can manage acute pain using pain managing modalities and a few body positions. But still, I would like to suggest you consult your doctor/ neurologist, as this stage is indeed a serious condition.

Any kind of movement or exercise is strictly prohibited and it can for the damage the already herniated disc.

Managing pain during the acute phase.

Acute pain and tenderness in the acute phase are so severe that a slightest of movement or twist can elicit a sharp shooting pain. Complete bed rest is advised to the sufferer.

If you have been prescribed with analgesics you should continue using it. In addition to the analgesics we can also administer heat treatment for the pain relief for this purpose hot fomentation would best work.

1. Rest

The rest is very important at this stage. Rest allows healing the damaged disc which otherwise would have been constantly under the stress. The patient is advised bed rest in the most comfortable position. It also helps in the reduction of acute tenderness around the lower back.

Resting position.

Acute sciatica sufferers should adopt a sleeping posture which makes them most comfortable.
But sleeping in a single posture for a long period is not possible and it is also not advisable.

Here is the guide to sleeping posture you can adapt. The best rest position would be the posture that gives you maximum comfort. I won't suggest using a pillow under the head, but you can try keeping it. If it feels comfortable than it ok to keep pillow below the head.

Below is the three rest position I would recommend. Choose the one which gives you maximum comfort.

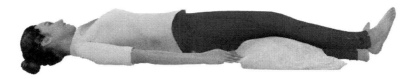

1: Sleep on your back with pillows under knee. Use a single or double layer of pillow depending on the comfort level.

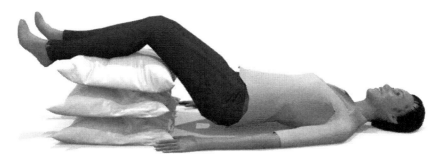

2: Sleep on your back with pillow as shown.

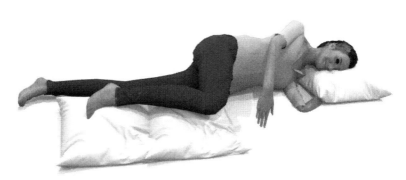

3: Side-lying with painful side upward and legs supported over the pillow

2. Heat treatment

In addition to the analgesics, heat treatment is advised for quick relief in pain. Heat treatment increases circulation, relieve congestion and relaxes muscular spasm.

Heat treatment can be given in many different ways
  1. Infrared radiation
  2. Shortwave diathermy
  3. Hot fomentation.

Infrared radiation and shortwave diathermy heating should be given under the supervision of a physiotherapist in a physiotherapy center. Since you are still in rest, I won't suggest you visiting the physiotherapy center.

So, what should you do at home?

At home, "hot fomentation" would be the best choice. Hot fomentation is actually an application of moist heat, which has a capability of deeper penetration thereby having more effectiveness.

Hot fomentation would best work after the application of pain balm. Apply a good pain balm thoroughly around the lower back on the painful region. After application of balm, leave it ideal for 10 minutes so that our body could absorb it.
After 10 minutes give hot fomentation over the same area for a minimum of 10 to 15 minutes.

Here I would like to mention the role of a physiotherapist. At any Physiotherapy Centre, the application of hot fomentation is done through a special instrument called as hydroculator.

Hydrocollator is electric heating equipment made up of steel. It is a chamber-like structure where it is filled with water. The chamber has an inbuilt heater which heats the water to the desired temperature.

Inside the water, the pads are kept for half an hour to an hour for observing the maximum heat.

These pads that somewhat resembles the weight cuff is filled with silica gel. Silica gels have the peculiar property of absorbing and retaining moisture for longer hence it retains the heat for longer period.

At home you can use a Turkish towel for hot fomentation it is very easy to use you can follow these steps to apply hot fomentation at your home.

1. Heat bowl of water on a gas stove to a temperature little less than boiling.
2. Optionally you can put 2 to 3 tablespoon of salt to make it more effective
3. Dip a towel into water and squeeze it firmly and apply it over the back
4. Repeat the process till water comes to the normal temperature.

How your physiotherapist can help you at this stage?

If you feel a little better, you must visit your physiotherapist. Though, your physiotherapist is the best person to decide which would most benefit you, here I am just presenting an overview of what you could expect there.

Please make a note that, this information is based on our own way of practicing at our center. You may find different approaches and instruments in your country. But, the basic treatment principle remains the same.

Short wave diathermy

Short wave diathermy has many advantages over other modes of heat treatment. The term diathermy means heating through or producing deep heating directly in the tissue of the body.

Oher heating device such as infrared lamps and electric heating pads produces more heat over the skin long before adequate heat has penetrated to the deeper tissues.

Another advantage of diathermy is that the treatment can be controlled precisely. Careful placement of the electrodes permits localization of the heat to the region to be treated. The amount of heat can be adjusted by means of parameters.

How this heating machine looks like.

A shortwave diathermy instrument consists of a machine with two points for output. From these points, two thick wire is connected and is attached to pads on the other end.

One pad releases an electromagnetic wave and another pad receives it. If our body parts come in between the pads, the wave passes through the body producing heat on the tissue

The heating of the tissues is carried out by high-frequency alternating current which has a frequency of 27.12 MHz and a wavelength of 11 meters. Currents of such high frequencies do not stimulate motor or sensory nerves nor do it produces any muscle contraction.

Application of pads.

The output of the SWD machine is connected to a metal electrode covered with rubber pads. Some machines have metal electrodes encased inside the glass disc. The pads/ disc are positioned over the painful body part (lower back). The electrodes never placed directly over the skin, usually, layers of a towel are interposed between the pad and surface of the body. For the disc, the little gap between skin is maintained.

The electrodes are placed such that it covers the whole the treating part and is sandwiched between them.

So, what's the principle behind this. Actually, the metal electrodes act as two plates of a capacitor and body tissues between as a dielectric. When the radiofrequency output is applied to the pads, the dielectric losses manifest themselves as heat in the intervention tissue.

Ultrasonic therapy

If you are curious about ultrasonic therapy (also called ultrasound), the very first point I would like to clarify is that it's not the ultrasound which is used for diagnostic purpose. People who first encounter ultrasonic therapy in our center often ask me out of curiosity, "what can you see about me on your machine?".

The therapeutic ultrasonic machine is used for treatment purpose and ultrasound imaging is used to take out images inside our body for diagnosing.

Note: ultrasonic therapy carries its own harmful effects, please do not try for yourself. Consult your physiotherapist if needed.

What is ultrasonic therapy?

Ultrasonic therapy is the treatment given using ultrasound waves emitted through the therapeutic ultrasonic machines.

Ultrasound wave, when given in a controlled condition has found to produce physiological effects in our body which cures many ailments. To understand its physiological effect we need to understand what is ultrasound waves and how it is produced?

Ultrasound is actually a sound wave whose frequency is higher than the frequency of the audible sound waves. An audible sound wave has a range of frequency which is audible to the human ear. The sound wave with frequency higher than the audible frequency is known as ultrasound wave.

Therapeutic ultrasound has a frequency between 0.7 and 3.3 megahertz (MHz).

Effects of ultrasonic therapy

The two important physiological effects of therapeutic ultrasound are thermal effect and non-thermal effect.

Thermal effect

The thermal effect or heating effect in the deep tissues is its most important physiological effect. It helps in the healing of tissue injuries that lie deeper by improving blood supply around the region.

Beneficial effects thought to arise from ultrasonically induced heating include(7):
1. Increase in the extensibility of collagenous structures such as tendons and scar tissue.
2. The decrease in joint stiffness.

3. Pain relief.
4. Changes in blood flow.
5. A decrease in muscle spasm and,
6. At high intensities, selective tissue ablation as achieved in focused ultrasound.

Non-thermal effect

Non-thermal mechanisms that can produce beneficial (therapeutic) changes in tissue may be cyclic or non-cyclic in nature(7).

- 'Micro-massage' effect: This is thought to be an effect due to the periodic nature of the sound pressure field.
- Acoustic streaming: Ultrasound waves produce a cavity that oscillates inside the intra- or extracellular fluid which is termed as acoustic streaming. Streaming may act to modify the local environment of a cell, leading, for example, to altered concentration gradients in the vicinity of an extracellular membrane. Streaming may account for the reported changes in the potassium and calcium content of cells following ultrasonic exposure.

IFT (Interferential Therapy)

Interferential therapy or IFT is an integral part of the physiotherapy treatment process. If you had been to any physiotherapy centre you might have observed physiotherapists connecting the patient to the machine through wires.

It produces a modified electric current which has found to be very effective in pain relief and gives a soothing or relaxing effect on the body part where it is applied.

What is IFT?

It is the production of beat frequency by the interference of two medium frequency currents.

To simplify it, two medium frequency currents are interfered with to produce a resulting high-frequency current. These two medium frequency current is of slightly different frequency so that when they interfere with each other they form constructive phase and destructive phase.
The following figure will clear it.

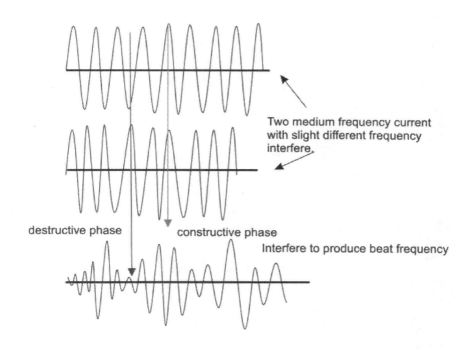

Two medium frequency current with slight different frequency interfere.

destructive phase   constructive phase

Interfere to produce beat frequency

Slight description of the machine.

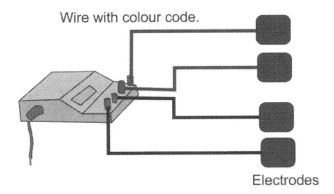

Wire with colour code.

Electrodes

IFT machine comes in two forms, one is for professional use and another is a portable one which can be used by any layperson with little training. Both have a similar design but vary in features.

IFT consists of the machine with the control button and a display panel from where the intensity of current supplied is controlled. It comes with four external wires with color code.

One pair (two wires) is a black color that forms one channel and another pair is of red color which forms the other channel. One end of the wire is connected to the machine and another end to electrodes. It is the electrodes that are directly connected to the body part where treatment is to be received. Electrodes can be made of metal or carbon rubber (nowadays vacuum electrode is gaining popularity).

To apply electrodes to the body, the electrodes are covered with a wet lint pad (special piece of cotton cloth made for this use). Some time gel is used in place of lint pad (note: the gel is used only for rubber electrode).

Effects of IFT.

1. Pain relief- It gives instantaneous pain relief and soothing effect.
2. Muscle spasm relief- The continuous contraction & relaxation of muscle creates muscle pump effect thereby improving the blood circulation. Its massage effect relaxes the spasmodic muscle.
3. Swelling reduction: Muscle pump effect helps drastically in improving the swelling.
4. Muscle relaxation.

Exercise in acute phase

In the acute phase, static exercises are more preferred over the dynamic exercises.
Why?

To understand this we first need to understand what is static and dynamic exercises.
Let me explain it with an example. Let us take two different exercises.

1. Sit on a long sitting position on a bed. Keep a pillow below the right knee and press it. Repeat this 10 times.
2. Sit on the edge of a table with legs hanging down. Now, slowly raise the right lower leg so as the right knee becomes fully straight.

One thing is common in both the exercise. Both exercises are the strengthening of the quadriceps muscle (muscle on the front of the thigh).

But, if you observe both the exercises closely, there is one major difference between them. In the first exercises, there is no movement of the leg or any other body part. In the second exercise, the knee is moving.

Did you get it? The first exercise in our example is a static exercise and the second exercise is a dynamic exercise.

So, what exercises have to be done in an acute stage?

Static exercise is important in this phase. But, we also allow slow controlled dynamic exercise for joints that are away from low back and are not causing any movement on back.
Below is the list of exercises which I commonly prescribe to our patient suffering from acute sciatica.

Static quadriceps contraction

This is a static exercise to strengthen the muscle on the front of the thigh.

- Sleep on your back with a pillow below the knee. If the condition permits, you can perform this exercise in a long sitting position also.
- Keep a pillow below the knee, You can also use the bedsheet/ towel roll.
- Press the pillow and count 1 to 5.
- Then release it slowly.
- Repeat it for a minimum of 30 times.
- Repeat the same process on the opposite knee.

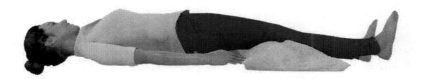

Ankle foot exercise

It is a dynamic exercise where the ankle is moving without causing any movement on the lower back.
In the same position as above, move the foot up and down. Repeat it on both the leg for a minimum of 30 times.

In prone lying raise your head

It is a dynamic exercise where the movement is occurring at the neck, away from the painful low back.

1. Lie down flat on your tummy.
2. Keep your hands by the side.
3. Slowly raise your head.
4. Repeat it for a minimum of 10 times.

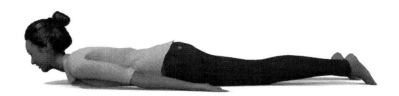

In prone lying contract your buttocks

A static exercise to strengthen the muscle of the buttocks
1. The starting position is the same as above. Lie down flat on your tummy.
2. Now, contract both the buttocks as if holding a piece of paper between buttocks.
3. Repeat this for a minimum of 30 times.

With the time your pain and tenderness around the lower back will reduce and after a few weeks, you should be able to at least come out of the bed and walk little distance on your own.

If there is no sign of improvement it is a red flag. You must be in constant touch with your neurosurgeon and proceed as suggested by them.

If everything goes fine, we enter into the next phase called the subacute phase.

.

Subacute Phase

"Look, you are not walking straight". Walking is painful but this is how home exercises and physiotherapy can help you.

n the subacute phase, most of the acute pain and tenderness are relieved. They can manage to move and ambulate with some pain. Acute sciatica improves to subacute phase, but it's not necessary that every subacute sciatica sufferers improves from acute sciatica stage. A person can directly be affected by subacute sciatica.

Remember, Mr. Sethy in the chapter "The story of Mr. Sethy", he is the best example of a sciatica sufferer directly entering into the subacute phase.

A subacute sciatica sufferer is no more bedridden, he can manage to get out of the bed, can carry out his daily chores, manage to walk but with some difficulty. He still complains of pain and numbness in the legs with a tingling sensation. Sometimes there may be a weakness in the legs and normal walking patterns may be affected by this weakness.

Clinical features of a subacute sciatica case.

1. By this stage, inflammation and severe pain subside.
2. Their main complaint is tingling sensation (electric shock-like feeling) on the back of the thigh and leg which increases with standing and walking.
3. Numbness over the sole of the foot. Numbness is mainly felt on the outer side of the foot.
4. Pulling sensation on the back of the leg that It starts from the buttocks, travels down the leg till the foot.

What can be done at home?

In subacute sciatica, reduced acuteness, tenderness allows some degree of movement, now one can focus on strengthening of the lower back muscles. A strong back muscle is important to support the back, it prevents pressure concentration over the degenerated lumbar disc.

One has to also take care of his posture and they must try to maintain a correct posture.
External back support by using lumbar braces also plays an important role in protecting the back and is extremely important during this phase. It plays an important role by supporting the back so that the weight of the upper trunk is evenly distributed over the support brace and there is less stress over the herniated disc.

The use of lumbar brace also becomes important as during walking there is a chance of recurrence of the hernia. It is highly advisable to use the brace during walking, standing or when driving in your car/ motorbike.

Managing pain in subacute phase

Though the pain reduces substantially by this phase, still sufferer complains of the slight pain with occasional flaring. So, it is advisable to continue the pain management program in this stage also.
For detail on each and every pain management topic, refer back to the acute stage chapter.

- Hot fomentation
- Application of pain balm.

You are also advised to attend physiotherapy on a regular basis. At your physiotherapy center these treatments you are expected to go through.

- Shortwave diathermy.
- Ultrasonic therapy.
- TENS (Transcutaneous Electrical Nerve Stimulation).
- Traction.

We have already discussed in detail the first three treatment options. You are advised to refer back to the chapter "Acute Phase".

Traction is an additional therapeutic process you may be given. Traction is a very effective and perhaps most popular physiotherapy treatment. It is a mechanical pull created over the lower back so that the reduced gap is re-widened giving way to a compressed nerve.

Traction has found to give almost instantaneous pain relief. So, let's dive deeper into this miraculous treatment machine.

Lumbar traction and its effect.

Every one of you must have experienced, if not experienced, must have seen/ heard of people taking traction for back pain. Traction not only relieves back pain without medication, but it can also cure complicated back pain cases such as sciatica and prolapsed disc.

Traction is an integral part of physiotherapy treatment. Just visit any physiotherapy center in your town, you are sure to spot a traction table. The physiotherapist also uses it for the treatment of other joint pain such as neck pain, knee pain.

What is lumbar traction?

Traction has been used as a medical intervention since antiquity. In modem time, James Cyriax popularized lumbar traction during the 1950s and 1960s as a treatment for disc protrusions. Today, traction continues to be a commonly employed modality for treating patients with back and leg pain(8).

It is a distraction force applied to the body part by the use of weight or mechanical pull.
We can define traction as a "distraction force applied over the vertebrae in an attempt to separate two vertebral bodies from each other. In lumbar spinal traction, the traction is applied over the lower back".

Effect of lumbar traction

There are three beneficial effects of traction as described by sir James Cyriax.
1. Distraction to increase the intervertebral space,
2. Tensing of the posterior longitudinal ligament to exert centripetal force at the back of the joint, and
3. Suction to draw the protrusion toward the center of the joint.
4. Other effects attributed to traction include the widening of the intervertebral foramen, flattening of the lumbar lordosis and distraction of the apophyseal joint.

The third effect of suction to draw the protrusion towards the center is very important in the treatment of disc protrusion.

Method of application of traction:

With time there is a significant improvement in the way the traction is applied. Slowly it has evolved towards a more automated and mechanical way, where the force of traction and its duration of application is under control. We can easily change the duration of traction applied and its force with the press of a button.

In older days traction was given using weight (gravity assisted). Weight such as sandbags or bricks were used to achieve traction for the lower back. The person was made to lie flat on the bed with a lumbar belt on, that comes fitted with hooks on the sides. A rope is hooked to both the side of the belt with another end of rope a calculated measure of weight is hanged.

One of the most important advantages of manual traction is its ease of use at home. However, it also carries its own disadvantages. Continuous traction for 20 to 30 minutes without break could result in increased pain and it is not recommended for severe back pain.

I personally never use continuous traction in my practice.

However, mechanical traction comes with both intermittent traction and static traction.
This motorized traction equipment changed the way traction is used in contemporary physiotherapy. Let us discuss the mechanical traction, its effect, and use.

The mechanical traction

Mechanical traction has the option for both continuous traction and intermittent traction.

Continuous traction produces muscle soreness. But what if it is interrupted by a short duration of relaxation?

For example, if the total duration of traction is 10 minutes, every 40 seconds of pull is interrupted by 10 seconds of relaxation period. This is possible by this mechanized traction.

Mechanized traction consists of a traction machine, a traction bed, one chest piece belt, and a low back piece belt. The image below is of a traction machine which is the most scientifically accepted traction machine of lumbar traction.

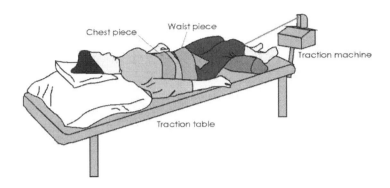

Traction at home.

Is it possible to get the benefit of traction at home?
Yes! It is possible. You can use the traction kit specially designed for home use. Just take care of how much weight /force you are using to apply traction. This traction is easily available in shops and also it is very easy to install. Just follow the installation procedure on the manual that comes with the product. Start with low weight and then progress further.

Exercises in subacute phase

I n the subacute phase of sciatica, the low back is capable to bear some stress. This gives us the opportunity to start the exercise and increase the stress-bearing capability of back.

Because of pain and lack of activity for longer period of time, the muscles around the back become weak. A weak muscle is incapable of holding the weight of the upper trunk thereby transferring all weight over the disc via the vertebral body.

Exercises help strengthen these muscles of the lower back. A strong muscle takes up most of the stress over it and distributes the stress evenly. This causes the release of excessive stress over the disc.

So let's start it get started with strengthening exercises.

Strengthening exercise

1: Bridging exercise.

1. Lye down on your back.
2. Keep both the hands by the side and bend both of your knees.
3. Then slowly lift your buttocks to its maximum.
4. Hold it for 10 sec and lower it down slowly (count 1 to 10)
5. Repeat this for a minimum of 30 times in a single session.

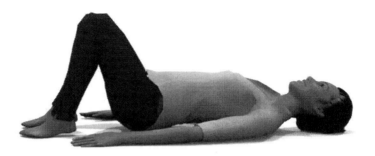

Starting position

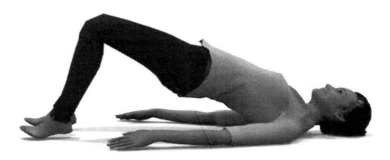

Target position

2: In prone chest raising.

1. Lye down on your tummy (supine lying) with the hands by the side.
2. Keeping your leg still, slowly raise your head and chest.
3. Raise to its maximum and hold it for 5 sec.
4. Then slowly lower yourself. Repeat it for minimum 10 times in a single session.

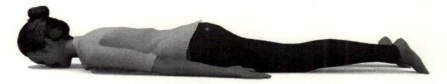

Starting position

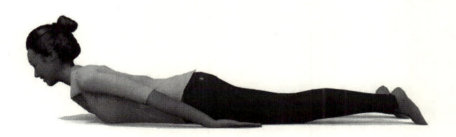

Target position

3: In prone lifting leg straight.

1. Again lye down on your tummy keeping both the hands by the side of your body.
2. Slowly raise your leg keeping the knee straight. Rise it to not more than 30 degrees of angle.
3. Hold it for 5 sec and lower it down slowly.
4. Repeat this for the opposite leg.
5. Do this on both legs alternately.
6. Repeat it for a minimum of 10 times in the single leg.

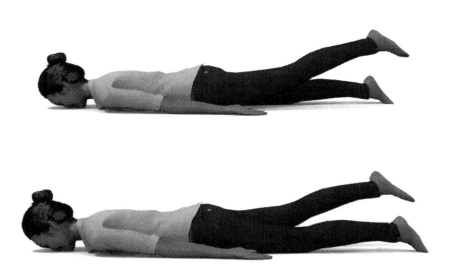

4: In prone lying lifting the leg and opposite hand alternately.

1. Come to the prone kneeling position as shown in the figure.
2. Raise one of your legs and the opposite hand. Elbow joint and knee joint should be as straight as possible.
3. For example, if the right leg is raised, the left hand should be raised.
4. Hold the position for 10 seconds (count 1 to 10) and then lower down slowly.
5. Repeat this process on the other side.
6. Do it alternately on both the side for a minimum of 30 times.

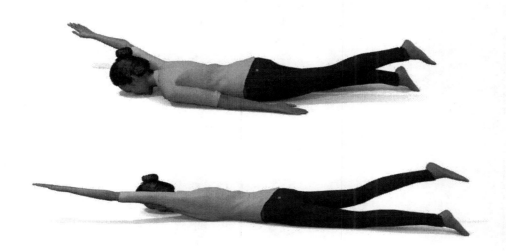

5: Cat and dog exercise.

1. Come to the prone kneeling position as shown in the figure.
2. Bow you back on the upper side and hold it for 5 seconds
3. Again bow your back to the lower side and hold for 5 seconds.
4. Repeat this process alternately on both sides for a minimum of 20 times.

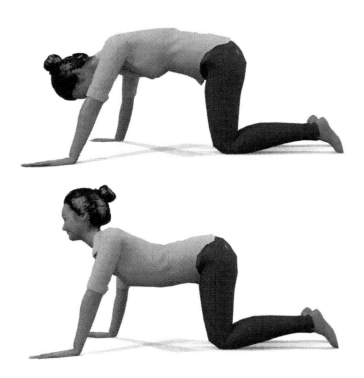

6: In prone kneeling lifting leg and opposite hand alternately

1. Start the exercise in prone kneeling position.
2. Raise one of your legs and the opposite hand. Elbow joint and knee joint should be as straight as possible.
3. For example, if the right leg is raised, the left hand should be raised.
4. Hold the position for 10 seconds (count 1 to 10) and then lower down slowly.
5. Repeat this process on the other side.
6. Do it alternately on both the side for a minimum of 30 times.

Piriformis stretching.

Piriformis is the muscle that is present on the sides of the buttock. Uln almost every back pain tightness and contracture of this muscle causes pain.
I prescribe this stretching exercise to almost all my back pain patients.

How to do it?
1. Lye down on your back with the hands by the side.
2. Keep both the legs straight.
3. Now, bend one of the knees and keep the foot over the opposite knee. A question might arise here, which knee? Ok, if you need to stretch your left knee then bend the left knee. It's that simple.
4. Hold the knee with both the hands and pull it towards the opposite shoulder in an oblique direction.
5. Hold it for a minimum of 60 sec (! minute) and then release it slowly.
6. Repeat the same exercise again on the other leg.
7. Do, it for 3 to 4 repetitions in a single session.

All the above exercises should be done at least twice daily. It would be wise if you do it once in the morning and again in the evening.

Rehabilitation phase

It's time to get back to your work. Pain is almost gone, but who can predict the future? Better get prepared with these precautions and exercises.

This is the last phase and it's the time to get back to your work. Most of the pain is significantly reduces by this time. You may have occasional complaints of pain and pulling sensation on the back of the thigh and leg when bending or sitting on the floor.

Walking has become much easier but running is still not advised. You can resume your normal routine but with some points of caution.

❏ Wear a lumbar belt during your routine morning walk.
❏ Never forget this belt while driving a motorbike or car.
❏ As far as possible avoid long distance travel.
❏ Avoid forward bending.
❏ Stay away from lifting heavyweight

The rehabilitation phase is all about precautions and exercises.
Repeat each and every exercises that we have discussed in the subacute phase but this time in a more rigorous way.
Increase the duration and count of all exercises.

Before we could once again move on to exercises part here are few important precautions and do's and don'ts of sciatica.

Precautions for sciatica sufferer

Sciatica sufferer needs to be very cautious. They have to be cautious during the daily chores so that they do not do an activity that is strictly contraindicated.
When going outdoor, always put your lumbar brace, it's a must thing if you are driving or going for a long journey. Although, a long journey but should be avoided altogether.

There is a list of "to do" and "not to do" points which you must adhere to it till you come out of the subacute phase.

So, here are some important precautions. Read it carefully, if possible discuss it with your physiotherapist and doctors.

1. Avoid flexion biased activities.
2. Adopt the correct way to reaching up to the floor.
3. Adopt the correct way of getting in and out of bed.

Let us discuss one by one in a detailed manner.

Avoid flexion (bending forward) biased activities.

Your doctors and physiotherapist must have advised you not to bend forward. Bending forward or to be more scientific, flexion activities increases the damage to the already damaged intervertebral disc.

There are lots of daily activity we perform it by bending ourself forward. It all happens subconsciously and it's not our fault. We are accustomed to doing it this way. But now, we need to change this.

I know it could be difficult, but be always careful and try to constantly remind yourself that "I have not to bend myself".

Here are the things you should avoid.

1. Bending forward
2. Sitting crossed leg sitting
3. Squatting.

All the above activity involves bending at the hip and lower back. These activities are to be avoided as it will further increase the disc bulge.

This could be understood with this diagram.

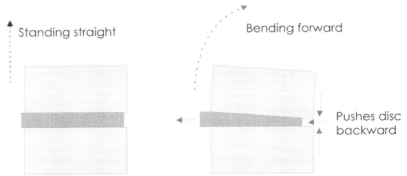

Standing straight

Bending forward

Pushes disc backward

A herniated disc when standing straight. Bending forward exerts destructive pressure which otherwise is harmless with normal disc.

In the diagram observe that how bending causes further pressure or already herniated disc only to aggravated the condition.

The correct way of picking up things from the floor.

If bending is contraindicated than how one could carry daily activity?

You might be asking yourself, what if:

1. I need to pick up a thing like a pen from the floor.
2. How would I reach under the bed to take a fallen piece of paper?
3. What if I need to lift my carry bag?

Yes it's impossible to avoid it, but, we can surely modify it to lessen the impact on our back

So, here is the correct way.
Consider a situation where you need to pick up a pen lying on the floor. What would be our usual way to accomplish this task?

1. The first diagram depicts the usual way which is to avoid.
2. The correct way is to bend yourself at knee and hip slowly lowering down and reaching upto the floor and get up the same way as you.

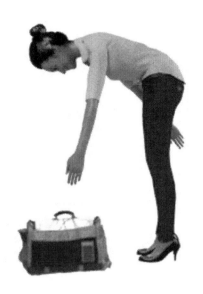

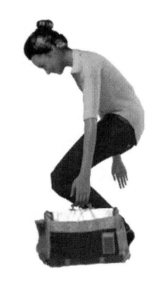

Gym ball exercise

Congratulations, if you have thoroughly followed the instructions of this book you are sure to lead a pain-free life hereafter. I understand how painful it was and it would indeed be a nightmare to suffering from it again. Coming out of sciatica is indeed like a coming to Heaven From Hell

However, there is a small word of caution from my side, there is a (low) chance of recurrence in the future. Though the chances of recurrence are very low, still we should not take a chance. I would like to advise you to continue a few important exercises for the rest of your life. Make it a part of your daily routine.

Doesn't it sound boring, the same boring exercises again and again? I know, this could really be boring and this is why in this chapter we going to discuss a different kind of exercises. And good thing is that it bears the same therapeutic effect and even it is a fun way of doing it that you will love it.

All you need is a gym ball.

Hey wait, I am not telling you to go to a gym. The exercises I am going to describe can easily be at home, you need a gym ball (also known as therapy ball) that is easily available at any sports shop.

I have a gym ball but does it fit my size

Gym ball comes three different shapes of spherical, oval and pear shape with various sizes.

- 18 inches (45cm)
- 22 inches (55cm)

- 26 inches (65cm)
- 30 inches (75cm)

Which size would best suit you? Most of the time 75 inches ball would best serve the purpose but if you would like to be specific there is a simple way to find it.

Sit on the inflated ball, come to a comfortable position and now look for your hip and knee. If the ball is of correct size then the hip and knee will be at 90 degrees of angle.

Try this with few different sizes and select the one that nearly gives you 90 degrees of angle to hip and knee.

See the figure below.

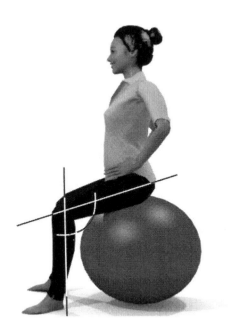

Now that we have found our gym ball let's go for exercise.

Forward and backward rocking.

1. Sit straight on the therapy ball.
2. Balance yourself, then forward rock your hip and backward rock alternately
3. Repeat this for a minimum of 20 times.

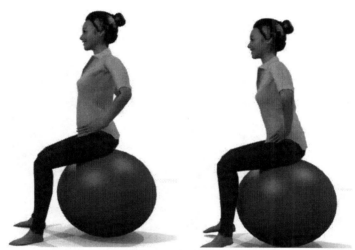

Backward rocking and Forward rocking

Sideways rocking.

A described above, sit straight on the ball and rock your pelvis sideways.

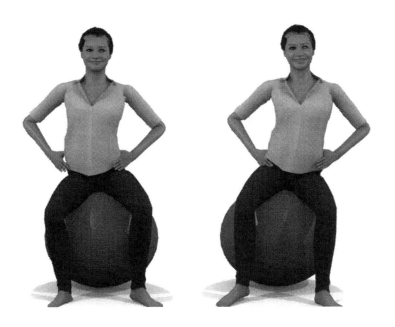

Left side rocking and Right side rocking

Bridging exercise.

1. Lie flat on your back
2. Keep the ball below the legs.
3. Position yourself so that your knee and hip joints remain in 90 degrees of angle
4. Slowly raise your back and hold the position for 5 seconds.
5. Repeat this for a minimum of 30 times.

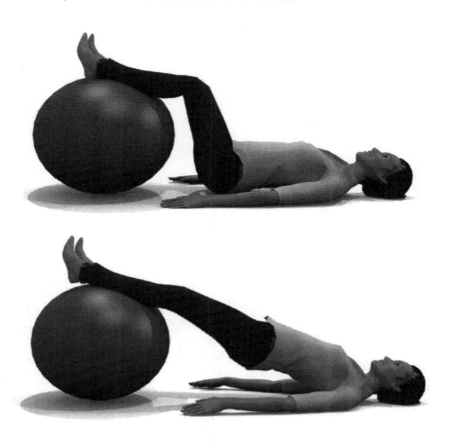

Straight leg raise in prone lying.

1. Come to the prone lying position.
2. Carefully slide the ball beneath your chest.
3. Now straighten your hip knee and elbow and balance yourself as shown in the figure.
4. Raise one of the legs and remain in the position for 5 seconds.
5. Raise the other leg and again hold for 5 seconds.
6. Repeat it alternately for a minimum of 30 repetitions.

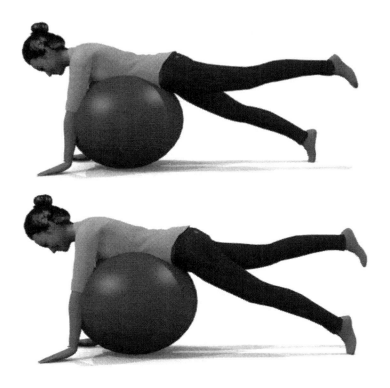

Straight leg raise and hand raise in prone lying.

1. Your starting position should be as described in the above exercise.

95

2. Do straight leg raise on the left side and simultaneously raise the opposite right side arm and forearm.
3. Hold this posture for 5 seconds.
4. Repeat it on the opposite side.
5. Repeat the exercises on alternate sides for a minimum of 30 times.

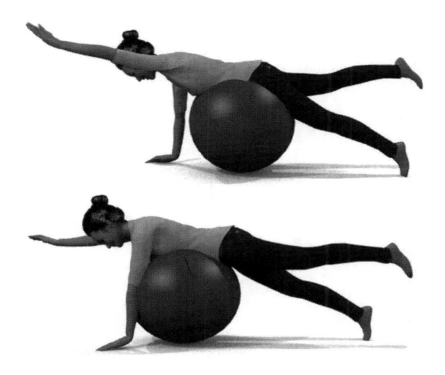

Side stretching exercise.

1. Lie down flat on your back and slide the ball below your leg.
2. Adjust yourself and then roll the ball onto one side.
3. Keep this position for 60 seconds.
4. Now slide the ball on the opposite side and hold for 6o seconds
5. Repeat 2 to 3 times on each side.

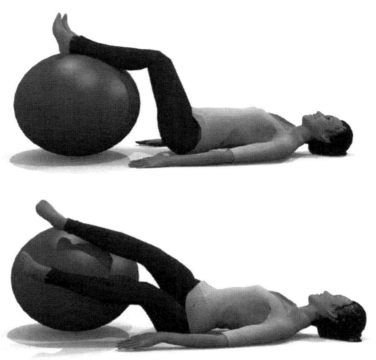

Electrical stimulation for pain called TENS

Remember that pin-pricking kind of electric shock your physiotherapist used to give you. Yes, we call this electric mode of treatment as TENS.

TENS stands for Transcutaneous Electrical Nerve Stimulation. It is given for pain relief in neurological cases like sciatica. TheTENS which you have been receiving at your physiotherapy Centre is given by a professional machine.

In the future, there may be a situation that pain may arise occasionally. It would be a wise decision if you keep a TENS machine handy with you.

A doubt may arise, how could I use this complicated machine for myself?

Your doubt is obvious but I have my answer ready. You don't need to use those complicated professional machines. Leave them for professionals only.

Because there is a portable model of TENS that is easily available in your local market.
This battery-operated tens machine is specially designed for personal use at home it is very easy to use.

And here I am going to teach you how to use it.

Parts of a portable TENS machine.

The TENS system consists of the main unit with all its control to increase or decrease the intensity or to change the program. It also consists of two outputs from where two wires come out and there are two electrodes attached to the other end of the wires.

The two electrodes come in direct contact with the body.

Follow these steps to apply it for your sciatica pain. Let us take the right side sciatica as an example.

1. Lie down flat on your tummy and expose your lower back.
2. Clean the right side lower back region and just below the calf muscles with the help of cotton and if possible cotton soaked in spirit.
3. Now place one electrode on the right side of the lower back and another electrode on the lower leg region just below the calf muscles. Hold it the electrodes in the place using straps or micropore tape.

This is the standard arrangement of the electrodes for sciatica pain, now slowly increase the intensity to the point where you can tolerate it. Remember the intensity should not beyond the tolerable range.

The duration of the stimulus stimulation could be 10 to 15 minutes and a maximum of 20 minutes. It should not go beyond 20 minutes, rather if needed you can apply it twice a daily.

The correct way of using a lumbar belt

The lumbar belt work as a support system for a weak painful back. It also has an important function in protecting low back from any movement and jerk.

I have seen many cases using a lumbar belt but they do not know the proper way of using it. So, here is a guide to using a lumbar belt in the correct way or a correct method.

Note: This method of using a lumbar belt is applicable in all kinds of lower back pain, so if you're having back pain (other than sciatica) you can follow simple tips.

Effects of using a lumbar belt.
- Supports sensorimotor function.
- Activate the muscular stabilization of the lumbar spine.
- Helps to relieve pain
- Reliefs the lumbar spine through increasing the intraabdominal pressure and external stabilization.

Size of the belt

The first thing about the lumbar belt is the correct size, a correct size lumbar belt snuggly fits your low back and give maximum support. But the wrong size will not give you the benefits of using it.

The lumbar belt comes in 5 different sizes.

❏ S for small.

- ❏ M for medium.
- ❏ L for large.
- ❏ XL for extra large.
- ❏ XXL for extra extra large.

Here is the step to find the correct size for yourself. Take an inch tape and measure the circumference of your waist. Note it down in a piece of paper and compare it with the table given below.

Size	(cm)	(inch)
S	70 - 80	27.6 - 31.5
M	80 - 90	31.5 - 35.4
L	90 - 100	35.4 - 39.4
XL	100 - 110	39.4 - 43.3
XXL	110 - 120	43.3 - 47.2

The proper way to wear a lumbar belt.

Many lumbar belts come with a contour that fits into the curves of the lower back. When using such a belt make sure that curves of belt fit with the curve of your back.

Some belts are manufactured simple and flat. Using this type of belt could be tricky. It could be confusing at which level of the back you should wear it.

Here is the proper way to judge the back level for a simple flat belt. First, try to locate the most painful point. It could be at the level of the hip or a little higher or just below the thorax.

Once you have successfully located it, take the belt and place the center of belt over the painful point. Make sure that the alignment of the belt should remain unaltered.

Afterwords

Slip disc (disc hernia/ disc bulge/ prolapsed intervertebral disc) is the major cause of sciatica. This book is oriented towards the treatment of sciatica due to a slipped disc.

But, there are many other uncommon causes that can not be ignored. They can be spinal canal stenosis, fibromyalgia, derangement of the sacroiliac joint, etc. In my 14 years of physiotherapy career, I have seen a most painful case which I would like to describe and end this book with.

A 35 years old nun suffering from subacute sciatica was referred to me. Although she had all the symptoms of sciatica, the real cause was different from what was diagnosed. It came into light after almost a year.

When she came to me, she was diagnosed with left side mild disc hernia with compression of neuronal structure. I planned my treatment program accordingly. After a week of treatment, she reported no significant improvement. Although she does reported momentary pain relief for a few hours immediately after treatment.

We continued with the treatment for almost 2 months without any significant result. With the time her pain aggravated after which she discontinued.

After one year she again came back to me to just report that she is fully cured. I went through all the treatment records and found that the actual cause was very different.

She actually had a uterine tumor. Tumor growth near to sciatic nerve caused its compression. The surgical removal of the tumor solved her pain.

Why I am mentioning this story (actually a real event)?

I just want to give this message. If your sciatica pain is not responding to these exercises or physiotherapy go to your doctor and discuss it with them. Your doctor could investigate the pain from a different angle.

With this, I end this book.

Wishing you all sciatica sufferer a speedy recovery.

About the author

Dr. Sunit Sanjay Ekka (PT) is a physiotherapist practicing for the last 14 years. He owns a successful physiotherapy center named "Physiofirst" at Rourkela, Odisha, India.

He holds a Bachelor's in Physiotherapy (BPT) from SVNIRTAR (Swami Vivekananda National Institute of rehabilitation and research), one of the prestigious Government physiotherapy schools of India.

Taking every pain and disability case as a challenge is his motto. Whatever he learns dealing with his patient, he shares it with the world through blog and e-books

He also owns a blog "www.physiosunit.com", where he shares everything he gets to learn from the patient. His knowledge and invaluable experience in the field is proving beneficial to many.

Email him: sunitekka@gmail.com
Join him: www.facebook.com/physiocapsule

References:

1. Mahadevan V. Anatomy of the vertebral column. Surg - Oxf Int Ed. 2018 Jul 1;36(7):327–32.
2. Stafford MA, Peng P, Hill DA. Sciatica: a review of history, epidemiology, pathogenesis, and the role of epidural steroid injection in management. BJA Br J Anaesth. 2007 Aug 17;99(4):461–73.
3. Ropper AH, Zafonte RD. Sciatica. N Engl J Med. 2015 Mar 25;372(13):1240–8.
4. Raj PP. Intervertebral Disc: Anatomy-Physiology-Pathophysiology-Treatment. Pain Pract. 2008 Jan 1;8(1):18–44.
5. Chang C, Jeno SH, Varacallo M. Anatomy, Bony Pelvis, and Lower Limb, Piriformis Muscle. In: StatPearls [Internet]. Treasure Island (FL): StatPearls Publishing; 2019 [cited 2019 Sep 28]. Available from: http://www.ncbi.nlm.nih.gov/books/NBK519497/
6. Roy BA. Piriformis Syndrome. ACSMs Health Fit J [Internet]. 2014;18(4). Available from: https://journals.lww.com/acsm-healthfitness/Fulltext/2014/07000/Piriformis_Syndrome.3.aspx
7. Haar G ter. Therapeutic ultrasound. European Journal of Ultrasound; 1999.
8. Pellecchia GL. Lumbar Traction: A Review of the Literature. J Orthop Sports Phys Ther. 1994 Nov 1;20(5):262–7.

BOOKS BY DR SUNIT

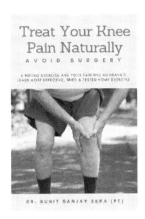

Treat Your Knee Pain Naturally

A wrong exercise and your knee pain will aggravate. Learn most effective, tried & tested home exercises for knee pain.

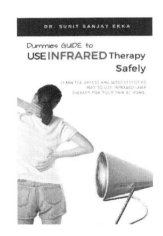

Dummies Guide to Use Infrared Therapy safely

Learn the safest and most effective way to use infrared therapy for your pain at home.

Manufactured by Amazon.ca
Bolton, ON

51435400R00065